5:2 DIET RECIPES

Delicious 30 MINUTE Fast Diet Recipes Under 500 Calories for Easier Fast Days

Gina Crawford

Evita Publishing, PO Box 306, Station A, Vancouver Island, BC V9W 5B1 Canada

IMPORTANT

The information in this book reflects the author's research, experiences, and opinions and is not intended to replace medical advice.

Before beginning this or any nutritional or exercise regimen, consult your physician to be sure it is appropriate for you. Ask for a physical stress test.

Table of Contents

Introduction

The 5:2 diet is a unique and powerful approach to dieting that can transform your health and weight for life! It is a modern phenomenon that is sweeping the nation with a new way of thinking about what the right way to diet really is.

The 5:2 diet focuses on intermittent fasting as a vehicle for weight loss and longevity. The benefits of fasting have been studied by scientists for years and they're research shows a strong correlation between fasting, life extension, better health, and weight loss.

5:2 Diet Recipes follows the recommended fast day eating schedule of the founder of the 5:2 diet Dr. Michael Mosley, who ate a light breakfast and dinner 12 hours apart on fast days.

In *5:2 Diet Recipes* you'll get sixty 30 minute fast day breakfast and dinner recipes that are quick, easy, and delicious. These low glycemic recipes are so tasty you'll forget you're fasting!

If you receive value from this book please consider posting a review on Amazon. Even a one or two line review is helpful and appreciated.

Chapter 1

What is the 5:2 Diet?

"Fasting is the first thing I've come across that I genuinely believe, if people were to take it up, could radically transform the nation's health."

Dr. Michael Mosley

The 5:2 diet, or *fast diet,* is a unique approach to dieting that uses intermittent fasting to promote weight loss and better health. It was popularized in 2012 by Dr. Michael Mosley, a British television journalist, producer, and science presenter.

Though the 5:2 diet itself is fairly new, the concept of fasting and the study of the benefits of fasting on human health are not. Some of the world's leading scientists have been studying the tremendous health benefits of fasting for over 20 years.

The 5:2 diet is unique in that it challenges our understanding of what the right way to diet really is. We've been taught to believe that in order to maintain a healthy lifestyle and lose weight it's important to eat regularly (six small meals a day), avoid getting hungry, consume low-fat foods, and exercise for a minimum of 30 minutes a day.

The 5:2 diet on the other hand, tells you to:

Fast on two non-consecutive days of the week by cutting your calorie intake to about one quarter of what it normally is (500 calories for women, 600 calories for men).

Eat what you want for 5 days a week.

Do a high intensity workout for ten minutes three times a week along with some strength training.

Why does the 5:2 diet work?

The human body was designed to fast

Human beings evolved at a time when feast or famine was the norm. Thousands of years ago, eating three to four meals a day was unheard of. People back then would kill something, eat it, and then eat nothing until they went out again to hunt their next meal.

This interim period of not eating caused the body to become stressed at a cellular level, but it was a good kind of stress that prompted the body to go into a repair and maintenance mode which ultimately made the body healthier and tougher. In science this is called hormesis.

This process is similar to what happens when you exercise. Muscles get torn and stressed but when you recover, you recover a lot stronger than before you exercised.

The 5:2 diet works because fasting on two non-consecutive days intentionally provokes good stress in the body and that promotes better health and weight loss.

You consume less calories

The 5:2 diet works because you consume only one quarter of your regular daily calories two days a week.

According to physics, that means you should expect to lose about one pound of fat per week.

When you first start the 5:2 diet, you will typically look like you've lost more than one pound per week because you'll be losing water.

As you continue with the diet you can expect to keep losing about one pound of fat per week without muscle loss.

It's not your typical diet

The 5:2 diet works because it doesn't involve the usual diet dread that comes with knowing that you've got eight weeks ahead of you of eating nothing but leaves and carrot sticks.

Because the 5:2 diet allows you to eat a chocolate bar if you want it, it actually lessons your temptation for it. Plus, learning to eat good sources of protein and vegetables on fast days helps you crave healthy foods more often.

High intensity workouts maximize your efforts

The effectiveness of high intensity workouts is a new evolving field of study. Scientists are changing the current view of exercise by proving that only three minutes of high intensity exercise per week can make a dramatic difference.

Pairing a high intensity workout with the 5:2 diet will boost your dieting efforts.

There's nothing complicated about it

The 5:2 diet is a straight-forward, easy to implement diet that does not involve awkward and lengthy rules, monotonous calorie counting, or deprivation.

It's a lifestyle

The 5:2 diet will help you lose weight but its long term health benefits will likely entice you to stick with it.

The 5:2 diet decreases your risk of a number of diseases including heart disease, cancer, and diabetes. It promotes a healthy, long, and energetic life.

Chapter 2

Why was the 5:2 Diet Created?

The 5:2 diet was created by Dr. Michael Mosley, a British (non-practicing) general physician. Mosley originally studied medicine with the intention of becoming a psychiatrist but upon graduation changed his focus to television. He went on to produce several science programs for the BBC that covered a wide range of topics from neuroscience to weight loss.

Mosley is well known for his programs that focus on medicine and biology, particularly his series on the workings of the human body, inside the human body.

In 1995 the British Medical Association named Dr. Michael Mosley, Medical Journalist of the Year.

In 2012, Dr. Mosley appeared in the BBC 2 Horizon documentary *Eat, Fast, Live Longer* which had a huge global response. Later that year he was credited with popularizing the 5:2 diet.

Why Dr. Mosley developed the 5:2 diet

Two years prior to popularizing the 5:2 diet, Mosley went to see his doctor for a routine checkup and was unexpectedly diagnosed with diabetes due to his extremely high blood sugar levels. He was also told that his cholesterol level was too high and that he had metabolic syndrome.

Though he didn't appear overweight on the outside he was fat on the inside with visceral fat. Visceral fat is stored in the abdominal cavity (stomach) around important internal organs like the pancreas, liver, and intestines. It can severely increase the risk of developing heart disease and diabetes.

Mosley's doctor wanted to start him on drugs in order to treat his illnesses, but Mosley declined because he was interested in seeing if there was a way to cure his condition without drugs. Shortly after Mosley started researching alternative healing methods he came across the concept of intermittent fasting.

With a keen interest in self-experimentation and testing dieting methods that seemed rather off the wall, he and the editor of the science branch of the BBC (Horizon) agreed to make a film in which he would test intermittent fasting on himself to see if it could improve his health.

At first he tried the regular dieting advice that he was taught as a doctor but it had no significant impact on his health. He then started a calorie restriction diet that involved eating a very small amount of calories every day. He personally found this plan quite difficult and almost impossible to maintain.

He then dove into intermittent fasting and began exploring the different ways in which intermittent fasting could be done. Some methods involved fasting for 24 hours or more. Others involved eating one low calorie meal once every two days.

After trying various methods of intermittent fasting, Mosley concluded that the methods he tried were too hard physically, psychologically, and socially, so he set out to devise his own method of intermittent fasting.

The 5:2 *fast diet* that Mosley designed was based on a number of different methods of intermittent fasting.

He decided to eat normally for five out of seven days and then do a modified fast on two non-consecutive days, cutting his caloric intake on the fast days to one quarter of his usual daily calories.

Dr. Mosley chose to fast on Mondays and Thursdays because he was inspired by the prophet Mohammed who told his followers to fast not only on a monthly basis for Ramadan, but also to cut their calories for two days a week, specifically on Mondays and Thursdays.

He stuck with what he termed the 5:2 diet for about 3 months and lost about 20 pounds of fat.

His body fat decreased from 28% to 20%, his blood glucose returned to normal, his cholesterol went down, and his blood pressure improved.

His program *Eat, Fast, Live Longer* that documented his experiences of turning his health around aired in the summer of 2012. It was extremely well received and immediately began to popularize the 5:2 diet.

For more information on the 5:2 diet see my *5:2 Diet for Beginners* book on Amazon.

Chapter 3

30 MINUTE
Fast Day Breakfast Recipes
Under 500 Calories

Remember to stay well hydrated through the day by drinking as much water, black tea and black coffee as you want.

Tomato Zucchini Bake with Eggs and Basil

196 calories per serving

Serves 2

Ingredients

Zucchini.....2 large, chopped into chunks

Cherry tomatoes.....200 grams, halved

Garlic.....2 cloves, crushed

Olive oil.....1 tablespoon

Fresh basil.....1 small handful, chopped

Eggs.....2

Salt and pepper.....to taste

Directions

Heat the olive oil in a non-stick pan then add the zucchini. Fry for about 5 minutes until the zucchini is soft. Add the tomatoes, garlic, salt, pepper and stir. Cook for a few minutes. Make two pockets in the mixture and crack the eggs into the pockets. Cover the pan and cook until the eggs are done, about 3 minutes. Top with fresh basil and serve.

Nutrition per serving

Calories....196

Carbohydrates.....7 grams

Protein.....12 grams

Fat.....13 grams

Fibre.....3 grams

Sugar.....6 grams

Salt.....0.25 grams

Portobello Mushroom and Spinach Egg Nest

127 calories per serving

Serves 4

Ingredients

Portobello mushrooms.....4 large

Spinach leaves.....2 large handfuls

Tomatoes.....2 sliced

Garlic.....4 cloves chopped, divided

Olive oil.....2 tablespoons, divided

Eggs.....4

Salt and pepper.....to taste

Directions

Preheat the oven to 200 degrees.

Place each mushroom in an oven safe dish. Top each mushroom with two tomato slices and one chopped garlic clove. Drizzle each with half a tablespoon of olive oil and season with salt and pepper. Bake for 10 minutes.

Place a colander in the sink. Add the spinach leaves to it. Pour boiled water over the spinach to wilt the spinach leaves. Squeeze out the excess water then add the spinach to each of the four dishes.

Make a nest in the tomato garlic topping on each mushroom. Crack an egg into it. Return to oven and cook for 8 minutes. Serve.

Nutrition per serving

Calories....127

Carbohydrates.....5 grams

Protein.....9 grams

Fat.....8 grams

Fibre.....3 grams

Sugar.....5 grams

Salt.....0.4 grams

Tomato and Basil Omelet

360 calories per serving

Serves 1

Ingredients

Tomato.....1 diced

Fresh basil.....1 small handful, chopped

Green onions.....2 finely chopped

Vegetarian cheddar.....1 tablespoon, grated

Eggs.....2

Olive oil.....2 tablespoons, divided

Salt and pepper.....to taste

Directions

Mix the tomato, basil, green onions, cheese and half the oil in a bowl with salt and pepper.

Heat the rest of the oil in a small pan and swirl the eggs around the pan. Cook until the eggs have partially set.

Add the tomato mixture over half the omelet. Fold and serve.

Nutrition per serving

Calories....360

Carbohydrates.....3 grams

Protein.....20 grams

Fat.....30 grams

Fibre.....1 gram

Sugar.....3 grams

Salt.....0.72 grams

Banana Strawberry Porridge with Cinnamon

266 calories per serving

Serves 4

Ingredients

Skim milk.....450 ml

Porridge oats.....100 grams

Bananas.....3 sliced into rounds

Cinnamon.....5 teaspoons, divided

Strawberries.....400 grams, sliced

Plain fat-free natural yogurt.....150 grams

Honey....4 teaspoons, divided

Directions

In a medium saucepan combine porridge oats, skim milk, half the bananas and 1 teaspoon of cinnamon. Stir and bring to a boil. Lower heat and cook for 5 minutes stirring constantly. Divide the mixture into four bowls and top each bowl with strawberries, the remaining banana, yogurt, one teaspoon of cinnamon and one teaspoon of honey. Serve.

Nutrition per serving

Calories....266

Carbohydrates.....53 grams

Protein.....12 grams

Fat.....2 grams

Fibre.....5 grams

Sugar.....34 grams

Salt.....0.24 grams

Breakfast Turkish Menemen

222 calories per serving

Serves 4

Ingredients

Red pepper.....1 medium, seeded and sliced

Chopped tomatoes.....1 - 14 ounce can

Yellow onions.....2 small, sliced

Fresh parsley.....1 small bunch, chopped

Plain Greek yogurt.....8 tablespoons

Garlic.....4 cloves, crushed

1 red chili, seeded and sliced

Eggs.....4

Sugar.....2 teaspoons

Olive oil.....2 tablespoons

Salt.....to taste

Directions

Heat the olive oil in a frying pan. Add the red pepper, onions, and chili. Cook until soft. Add the tomatoes and sugar. Cook until the liquid has reduced. Season with salt.

Create four pockets in the mixture then crack the eggs into each pocket. Cover and cook on low until the eggs have set.

Mix the yogurt together with the garlic.

Remove the eggs from the pan and sprinkle each serving with fresh parsley.

Top each serving with two tablespoons of the yogurt garlic mix. Serve.

Nutrition per serving

Calories....222

Carbohydrates.....12 grams

Protein.....12 grams

Fat.....15 grams

Fibre.....3 grams

Sugar.....9 grams

Salt.....0.39 grams

Crème Fraîche Ham with Leeks and Cheese

295 calories per serving

Serves 4

Ingredients

Cooked ham.....8 medium cut slices

Leeks.....8 use the white part only

Cheddar cheese.....1 small handful, grated

Crème Fraîche.....6 tablespoons

Dijon mustard.....2 tablespoons

Salt.....to taste

Directions

Preheat the oven to 250 degrees. Cook the leeks in boiling water until soft. Drain and cool.

Wrap each leek in one slice of ham and place into a baking dish. Mix the cheese in a bowl with the crème fraîche, mustard and salt.

Spread the cheese mixture over the wrapped leeks and bake for 15 minutes until bubbling and light brown. Serve.

Nutrition per serving

Calories....295

Carbohydrates.....6 grams

Protein.....20 grams

Fat.....21 grams

Fibre.....3 grams

Sugar.....0 grams

Salt.....2 grams

Spinach and Zucchini Ricotta Frittata

211 calories per serving

Serves 4

Ingredients

Eggs.....6

Zucchini.....2 peeled and sliced

Spinach leaves.....2 large handfuls

Ricotta cheese.....125 grams

Dried red chili flakes.....1 teaspoon

Yellow onion.....1 small, sliced

Olive oil.....1 tablespoon

Salt.....to taste

Directions

Heat the olive oil and onion on a large frying pan.

When the onion is soft, add the chili flakes and zucchini and cook for 5 minutes.

Place a colander in the sink. Add the spinach leaves to it. Pour boiled water over the spinach to wilt the spinach leaves. Squeeze out the excess water and scatter the spinach onto the pan. Top with ricotta cheese.

Set the oven to broil. Beat the eggs and season with salt. Pour the eggs into the pan and cook until the eggs have partially set.

Place the egg mixture in the oven on broil and cook through. Serve.

Nutrition per serving

Calories....211

Carbohydrates.....6 grams

Protein.....15 grams

Fat.....15 grams

Fibre.....3 grams

Sugar.....5 grams

Salt.....0.5 grams

Creamy Mushroom and Basil Omelet

196 calories per serving

Serves 2

Ingredients

Tomatoes.....2 halved

Low-fat cream cheese.....2 tablespoons

Fresh basil leaves.....1 tablespoon, chopped

Shiitake mushrooms.....300 grams, sliced

Fresh chives.....1 tablespoon, chopped

Unsalted butter.....1 teaspoon

Eggs.....3

Water.....2 tablespoons

Salt and pepper.....to taste

Directions

Set the oven to broil. Place the tomato halves under broil on a piece of foil turning occasionally. When the tomatoes are grilled remove them from the heat then dice them. Set aside.

Mix the eggs, chives, water, salt, and pepper in a bowl. Set aside.

Heat a pan over medium heat then add butter to it. Add the mushrooms and cook for 5 minutes until soft. Remove from pan, cover and set aside. Leave the pan on the heat.

Add the egg mixture to the hot pan and swirl until eggs have partially set. Add the mushrooms, cream cheese, tomatoes, and basil to half the omelet. Fold the omelet and serve.

Nutrition per serving

Calories....196

Carbohydrates.....4 grams

Protein.....14 grams

Fat.....14 grams

Fibre.....3 grams

Sugar.....4 grams

Salt.....0.5 grams

Flaxseed and Apple Porridge

236 calories per serving

Serves 4

Ingredients

Porridge oats.....100 grams

Skim milk.....500 ml

Gala apples.....2 peeled and grated

Ground cinnamon.....2 tablespoons

Flaxseeds.....2 tablespoons

Plain Greek yogurt.....8 tablespoons, 2 tablespoons for each serving

Honey.....4 teaspoons, drizzle 1 teaspoon on top of each serving

Directions

In a medium saucepan, add the milk, oats, cinnamon and apples together and stir. Bring to a boil then lower the heat and cook for 4 minutes stirring constantly. Add the flaxseeds then divide the mixture into four bowls.

Top each with yogurt and honey. Serve.

Nutrition per serving

Calories....236

Carbohydrates.....29 grams

Protein.....12 grams

Fat.....6 grams

Fibre.....6 grams

Sugar.....15 grams

Salt.....0.2 grams

Tarragon and Chives Sunshine Omelet

396 calories per serving

Serves 1

Ingredients

Unsalted butter.....2 tablespoons

Freshly grated parmesan.....1 teaspoon

Fresh tarragon.....3 tablespoons, chopped

Fresh chives.....3 tablespoons, chopped

Gruyère cheese.....3 tablespoons, grated

Eggs.....3

Salt and pepper.....to taste

Directions

Heat a pan on medium heat then add the unsalted butter.

In a bowl, mix the eggs together with the parmesan, tarragon, chives, salt, and pepper. Pour the egg mixture into the pan and swirl.

When the eggs have partially set, add the cheese. Cook for 3 minutes then fold. Serve.

Nutrition per serving

Calories....396

Carbohydrates.....0 grams

Protein.....24 grams

Fat.....33 grams

Fibre.....0 grams

Sugar.....0 grams

Salt.....0.95 grams

Meaty Breakfast Bake with Fresh Chives

349 calories per serving

Serves 4

Ingredients

Italian sausage.....4 - 130 gram links, chopped into rounds

Bacon.....4 strips, diced

Eggs.....6

Cherry tomatoes.....8 halved

Button mushrooms.....1 large handful, sliced

Fresh chives.....1 tablespoon, chopped

Olive oil.....2 tablespoons

Seasoning salt.....to taste

Directions

Set the oven to broil.

Heat the oil in a pan on medium heat. Add the sausage and bacon to the pan and cook until the sausages have cooked through and the bacon is crisp. Remove from pan and set aside. Add the mushrooms and cook for 3 minutes.

Put the sausage and bacon back into the pan with the mushrooms.

Crack the eggs into a bowl and season with the salt. Whisk the eggs then add them to the pan with the sausage, bacon and mushrooms. Swirl to coat the pan. Add the tomatoes and chives then place the pan in the oven to broil for 2 minutes until set.

Cut into wedges. Serve.

Nutrition per serving

Calories....349

Carbohydrates.....4 grams

Protein.....25 grams

Fat.....26 grams

Fibre.....1 gram

Sugar.....2 grams

Salt.....2.27 grams

Cilantro Tomato Egg Extravaganza

340 calories per serving

Serves 2

Ingredients

Cherry tomatoes.....2 - 400 gram containers

Cilantro.....1 small bunch, chopped, divided

Red onion.....1 small handful, chopped

Garlic.....2 cloves, chopped

Eggs.....4

Sugar.....1 teaspoon

Olive oil.....1 tablespoon

Chili pepper.....1/4 teaspoon

Pumpernickel bread.....2 slices

Directions

Heat the oil in a pan. Add the chili pepper, garlic, red onion and half the cilantro. Cook for 5 minutes until soft. Stir in tomatoes and sugar and let the mixture come to a boil.

Make four pockets in the mixture and crack an egg into each pocket. Cover with lid then cook on low heat for 6 minutes until eggs are set. Top with remaining cilantro and serve with one slice of toasted pumpernickel bread.

Nutrition per serving

Calories....340

Carbohydrates.....21 grams

Protein.....21 grams

Fat.....20 grams

Fibre.....0 grams

Sugar.....17 grams

Salt.....1.25 grams

Mushroom Cheddar Omelet with Fresh Parsley and Sweet Oven Chips

391 calories per serving

Serves 1

Ingredients

Olive oil.....1 tablespoon

Button mushrooms.....1 cup, sliced

Vegetarian cheddar.....2 tablespoons, grated

Fresh parsley.....1 small handful, chopped

Sweet potato.....1 medium, cut into long strips

Eggs.....2

Salt and pepper.....to taste

Directions

Heat the oil in a pan over medium heat. Add the mushrooms and cook until soft. Remove the mushrooms from the pan and place them into a bowl.

Add the cheese and parsley to the bowl and mix.

Heat the pan once more and add the eggs. Swirl the eggs and cook them until they have partially set.

Place the mushroom mixture on half the omelet. Fold and serve with sweet oven chips.

Sweet oven chips

Place the sweet potato strips on a baking pan, drizzle with oil and season with salt and pepper. Place them in the oven at 300 degrees. Bake until soft.

Nutrition per serving

Calories....391

Carbohydrates.....0.3 grams

Protein.....22 grams

Fat.....33 grams

Fibre.....0.7 grams

Sugar.....0.2 grams

Salt.....0.9 grams

Minty Goat Cheese Frittata

306 calories per serving

Serves 4

Ingredients

Frozen peas.....300 grams

Skim milk.....splash

Goat cheese.....100 gram log. Cut 4 medium thick slices and crumble the rest.

Fresh mint.....2 tablespoons, chopped

Eggs.....8

Olive oil.....2 tablespoons

Salt and pepper.....to taste

Directions

Preheat the oven to 300 degrees.

Boil the peas in a pot of water until soft. Drain.

Beat the eggs in a bowl with salt and pepper, a splash of milk, the crumbled goat cheese, peas and fresh mint.

Spread the olive oil on an ovenproof shallow pan. Pour the egg mixture into the pan and bake in oven for about 8 minutes or until the eggs are almost cooked.

Top with the four slices of goat cheese then place the egg mixture under broil. Bake until the eggs have set and the cheese is bubbling and golden. Serve.

Nutrition per serving

Calories....306

Carbohydrates.....8 grams

Protein.....25 grams

Fat.....20 grams

Fibre.....4 grams

Sugar.....2 grams

Salt.....0.74 grams

Skinny-Minnie Tomato and Ham Omelet

206 calories per serving

Serves 2

Ingredients

Extra-lean ham.....5 medium cut slices, shredded

Green onions.....2 chopped, keep the white part of the green onion separate from the green part

Reduced-fat cheddar cheese.....2 tablespoons

Red pepper.....1 seeded and diced

Eggs.....2 whole eggs

Egg whites.....3

Olive oil.....1 teaspoon

Tomatoes.....2 sliced to serve

Salt and pepper.....to taste

Directions

Mix the eggs and egg whites together along with some salt and pepper. Set aside.

Heat the oil in a medium pan and cook the red pepper for 3 minutes. Add the white parts of the green onion and cook for 1 minute. Add the egg mix and cook over medium heat until partially set.

Sprinkle with ham and cheddar cheese and continue cooking until the eggs have set. Top with the tomato and green part of the green onions.

Nutrition per serving

Calories....206

Carbohydrates.....5 grams

Protein.....21 grams

Fat.....12 grams

Fibre.....1 gram

Sugar.....5 grams

Salt.....1.21 grams

Greek Sweet Porridge

175 calories per serving

Serves 1

Ingredients

Porridge oats.....1 handful

Skim milk.....350 ml

Plain Greek yogurt.....2 tablespoons, divided

Honey.....2 teaspoons, divided

Salt.....to taste

Directions

Place the porridge oats in a saucepan along with the milk and season with some salt. Bring to a boil then simmer for 4 minutes stirring occasionally.

Allow the porridge to stand for about 2 minutes before serving.

Pour into bowls and top with yogurt and honey.

Nutrition per serving

Calories....175

Carbohydrates.....25 grams

Protein.....10 grams

Fat.....5 grams

Fibre.....3 grams

Sugar.....0 grams

Salt.....0.24 grams

Spinach and Tomato Bake

114 calories per serving

Serves 4

Ingredients

Spinach leaves.....284 gram bag

Chopped or diced tomatoes.....1 - 400 gram can

Chili flakes.....1 teaspoon

Eggs.....4

Salt and pepper.....to taste

Directions

Preheat the oven to 250 degrees.

Place the spinach in a colander and pour boiled water over it to wilt the spinach leaves. Squeeze out the excess water. Divide the spinach between four oven safe dishes.

Mix the chili flakes, tomatoes, and salt and pepper together and add to the four spinach dishes. Create a well in the centre of the vegetable mixture and crack an egg into it. Bake for 12 minutes or until the eggs have set. Enjoy!

Nutrition per serving

Calories....114

Carbohydrates.....3 grams

Protein.....9 grams

Fat.....7 grams

Fibre.....2 grams

Sugar.....2 grams

Salt.....0.43 grams

Pear, Walnut and Cinnamon Porridge

341 calories per bowl

Serves 1

Ingredients

Porridge oats.....3 tablespoons

Water.....250 ml

Plain low-fat natural yogurt.....2 tablespoons

For the topping:

Pear.....1 sliced with skin

Walnut pieces.....1/4 cup

Cinnamon.....1 teaspoon

Directions

Combine the water and porridge oats in a saucepan over medium heat. Cook until bubbling and thick. Stir in the yogurt. Remove from the pan and place in a bowl. Top with pear, walnut pieces and cinnamon. Serve.

Nutrition per serving

Calories....341

Carbohydrates.....41 grams

Protein.....16 grams

Fat.....12 grams

Fibre.....8 grams

Sugar.....27 grams

Salt.....0.4 grams

Very Berry Good Omelet

264 calories per serving

Serves 1

Ingredients

Cottage cheese.....100 grams

Strawberries, blueberries and raspberries ....250 grams

Cinnamon.....1 teaspoon

Skim milk.....1 tablespoon

Egg.....1

Grape seed oil.....1/2 teaspoon

Directions

Beat the egg in a bowl with the milk and cinnamon.

Heat the oil on a pan then add the egg mixture, swirling to cover the pan. Cook until golden underneath. Do not fold.

Plate and top with cottage cheese and berries.

Roll up the omelet and serve.

Nutrition per serving

Calories....264

Carbohydrates.....18 grams

Protein.....21 grams

Fat.....12 grams

Fibre.....4 grams

Sugar.....16 grams

Salt.....1 gram

Cranberry Apricot Power Bar

78 calories per slice

Makes 14 slices

Ingredients

Dried apricots.....150 grams

Sesame seeds.....25 grams

Dried cranberries.....15 grams

Chia seeds.....1 tablespoon

Sunflower seeds.....1 tablespoon

Rolled oats.....40 grams

Boiling water.....150 ml

Desiccated coconut.....50 grams

Hemp protein powder.....3 tablespoons

Directions

Combine the apricots, boiling water, and oats in a food processor and purée. Transfer the mixture to a bowl.

Toast the coconut, sesame seeds, and sunflower seeds in a pan over low heat. Add to the apricot mixture.

Add the cranberries, chia seeds, and hemp protein powder to the apricot toasted seed mixture and combine into a thick paste.

Roll the mixture into a log on a sheet of plastic wrap. Wrap tightly then place in the fridge to chill. Cut and serve.

Nutrition per serving

Calories....78

Carbohydrates.....8 grams

Protein.....3 grams

Fat.....4 grams

Fibre.....3 grams

Sugar.....5 grams

Salt.....0 grams

Roasted Red Pepper, Artichoke and Basil Soufflé

275 calories per serving

Serves 4

Ingredients

Artichoke hearts.....1 – 6 ounce jar, drained and chopped

Roasted red pepper.....1 – 12 ounce jar, drained and chopped

Parmesan cheese.....4 tablespoons, divided

Fresh basil.....4 tablespoons, chopped

Eggs.....5 - separate the yolk from the whites

Whole eggs.....2

Butter.....1 tablespoon

Olive oil.....1 tablespoon

Salt and pepper

Directions

Set the oven to broil. Beat the egg yolks and two whole eggs together in a bowl. Use an electric whisk to beat the egg whites in a separate bowl. Add the egg whites to the yolks and combine carefully. Fold in the basil, roasted red pepper, artichokes, half the cheese, salt, and pepper.

Heat the butter and oil on a pan over medium heat. Add the egg mixture and spread over the pan evenly. Cook until it is lightly brown underneath. Sprinkle the remaining cheese on top then place the pan under broil and cook for 2 minutes. Cut the omelet into wedges. Serve.

Nutrition per serving

Calories....275

Carbohydrates.....2 grams

Protein.....19 grams

Fat.....21 grams

Fibre.....1 gram

Sugar.....1 gram

Salt.....1.01 grams

Greek Salad Style Omelet

371 calories per serving

Serves 4

Ingredients

Red onion.....1 cut into wedges

Feta cheese.....1 small handful, crumbled

Fresh parsley.....1 handful, chopped

Tomatoes.....3 chopped

Eggs.....10

Black olives.....2 tablespoons, pitted

Olive oil.....2 tablespoons

Salt and pepper

Directions

Set the oven to broil.

Whisk the eggs in a bowl with fresh parsley, salt, and pepper.

Heat the oil in a pan then fry the onion for 4 minutes until lightly brown. Add the olives and tomatoes and cook until soft.

Lower the heat to medium and add the eggs to the pan. Cook for about 2 minutes. Add the feta cheese then place the pan under broil for 5 minutes until the omelet is puffy and golden.

Cut the omelet into wedges and serve.

Nutrition per serving

Calories....371

Carbohydrates.....5 grams

Protein.....24 grams

Fat.....28 grams

Fibre.....1 gram

Sugar.....0 gram

Salt.....2 grams

Mascarpone Winter Fruit Breakfast Salad

192 calories per serving

Serves 6

Ingredients

Dried fruit mix (pears, figs, apricots, prunes, cranberries).....600 grams

Water.....24 ounces

Earl Grey tea bag.....1

Vanilla pod.....1 split lengthwise

Lemon.....1 tablespoon of juice

Honey.....3 tablespoons

Mascarpone.....1 tablespoon per serving

Directions

Combine the dried fruit mix and water in a saucepan over medium heat. Add the vanilla and honey and bring to a boil. Stir. Lower heat and simmer for about 10 minutes until the texture is syrupy.

Remove the saucepan from the heat and stir the tea bag in. Let the tea bag infuse the dried fruit for about 10 minutes.

Discard the vanilla pod and tea bag. Transfer the fruit mix and water to a bowl and top with lemon juice. Stir then cover and chill.

Top with one tablespoon of mascarpone per serving.

Nutrition per serving

Calories....192

Carbohydrates.....46 grams

Protein.....3 grams

Fat.....1 gram

Fibre.....6 grams

Sugar.....6 grams

Salt.....0.07 grams

Spiced Poached Pears with Orangey Yogurt

131 calories per serving

Serves 4

Ingredients

Pears.....4 halved and cored

Fresh cranberries.....1 handful

Cranberry jelly.....1 tablespoon

Honey.....1 tablespoon

Spiced tea bags.....2 (Apple Cinnamon flavored tea bags work great!)

Sugar.....2 tablespoons

Plain natural yogurt....1 cup

Orange juice.....4 ounces

Water.....16 ounces

Directions

Mix the yogurt and orange juice together in a bowl and set aside.

Combine the jelly, sugar, honey, and tea bags in a saucepan with water and bring to a boil. Stir. Add the pears then cover and simmer for 12 minutes until pears are tender.

Remove the pears and set aside. Increase the heat and add cranberries to the water. Boil until the water becomes syrupy. Remove the tea bags.

Plate the pears and pour the warm syrup over top with the orangey yogurt mixture.

Nutrition per serving

Calories....131

Carbohydrates.....34 grams

Protein.....1 gram

Fat.....0 grams

Fibre.....4 grams

Sugar.....34 grams

Salt.....0.02 grams

Sun-Dried Tomato and Feta Omelet

266 calories per serving

Serves 1

Ingredients

Sun-dried tomatoes.....1 – 7 ounce jar, drained and chopped

Feta cheese.....1 small handful, crumbled

Eggs.....2 whisked

Olive oil.....1 tablespoon

Salt and pepper

Directions

Heat the olive oil in a pan. Whisk the eggs in a bowl with salt and pepper then add them to the pan. Swirl the pan to coat.

When the eggs have partially set sprinkle the tomatoes and feta over half the omelet. Fold. Cook for another minute and serve.

Nutrition per serving

Calories....266

Carbohydrates.....5 grams

Protein.....18 grams

Fat.....20 grams

Fibre.....1 grams

Sugar.....4 grams

Salt.....1.8 grams

Fiber Blast

124 calories per serving

Makes about 18 breakfast bowls.

You can store this nutritious breakfast cereal in an airtight container for up to two months.

Ingredients

Wheat germ.....250 grams

Dark raisins.....100 grams

Jumbo oats.....300 grams

All Bran.....100 grams

Flax seeds.....50 grams

Apricots.....150 grams, cut into chunks

Brown sugar.....1 teaspoon per serving

Directions

Mix all the ingredients together in a large bowl.

When ready to serve, pour some of the mixture into a bowl and serve with milk.

Top with half an unpeeled diced apple.

Nutrition per serving

Calories....124

Carbohydrates.....23 grams

Protein.....4 grams

Fat.....3 grams

Fibre.....3 grams

Sugar.....1 gram

Salt.....0.16 grams

Pistachio and Grapefruit Morning Salad

107 calories per serving

Serves 2

Ingredients

Pink grapefruit & white grapefruit.....1 of each

Pistachio nuts.....2 teaspoons, divided

Agave nectar.....2 tablespoons, divided

Directions

Divide the grapefruit segments between two bowls and top with pistachios and agave nectar.

Nutrition per serving

Calories....107

Carbohydrates.....21 grams

Protein.....2 grams

Fat.....1 gram

Fibre.....2 grams

Sugar.....12 grams

Salt.....0 grams

Apricot, Orange and Grapefruit Wake Up Salad

83 calories per serving

Serves 4

Ingredients

Pink grapefruit.....2 segmented

Fresh apricots.....4 sliced

Oranges.....4 segmented

Honey.....1 tablespoon

Directions

Mix all the ingredients together in a large bowl.
Serve.

Nutrition per serving

Calories....83

Carbohydrates.....18 grams

Protein.....2 grams

Fat and salt.....0 grams

Fibre.....4 grams

Sugar.....18 grams

Chapter 4

30 MINUTE
Fast Day Dinner Recipes
Under 500 Calories

The job of fasting is to supply the body with the ideal environment to accomplish its work of healing.

Joel Fuhrman, M.D.

Thai Roasted Chicken with Minty Mango Apple Salad

275 calories per serving

Serves 2

Ingredients

For the chicken:

Boneless chicken breasts.....2 – 4 ounce pieces with skin

Fresh ginger.....3 inches, grated

Shallots.....3 halved

Juice and zest of 1 lime

Sunflower oil.....2 teaspoons

Salt....1 teaspoon

Fish sauce.....1 teaspoon

For the salad:

Mango.....1/2 peeled and cut into thin sticks

Fresh mint.....1/2 bunch, leaves picked

Red apple.....1 cut into thin sticks

Green onions.....3 sliced

Cilantro.....1/2 a small bunch, leaves picked

Sugar.....1/4 teaspoon

Salt.....to taste

Directions

Finely chop the shallots in a food processor. Add the ginger, lime zest, and salt and process to a chunky paste. Remove and put the paste in a frying pan with the oil. Fry for 2 minutes.

Heat the oven to 250 degrees. Stuff the shallot ginger paste under the skin of the chicken and roast for 15 minutes until the chicken is golden and cooked through.

For the salad, mix all the ingredients together and set aside.

Remove the chicken from the roaster. Place the roaster on the oven and add the cilantro, a splash of fish sauce, and the remaining lime juice to it. Scrape the chicken bits up to make a sauce.

Plate the chicken. Pour the sauce over the chicken and serve with the minty mango apple salad.

Nutrition per serving

Calories.....275

Carbohydrates.....22 grams

Protein.....33 grams

Fat.....7 grams

Fibre.....4 grams

Sugar.....20 grams

Salt.....0.8 grams

Smoked Salmon and Prawns with Crème Fraîche and Honey Lime Vinaigrette

266 calories per serving

Serves 2

Ingredients

Smoked salmon.....4 – 150 gram slices

Cooked prawns.....10 large, peeled with tails on

Horseradish.....1 teaspoon

Crème Fraîche.....1 tablespoon

For the salad:

Leafy green lettuce.....2 handfuls

Fresh ginger.....1/2 teaspoon, grated

Juice and zest of ½ a lime

Honey.....1 teaspoon

Olive oil.....4 tablespoons

Salt and pepper

Directions

Combine the horseradish, crème fraîche, salt, and pepper.

For the dressing, whisk the lime zest, lime juice, ginger, honey, salt, pepper, and olive oil together.

Toss the lettuce with the dressing then place it on a serving plate. Drizzle the remaining dressing on top and around the plate.

Place the prawns and smoked salmon on top of the lettuce then drizzle the horseradish mixture on top of the meat. Serve.

Nutrition per serving

Calories.....266

Carbohydrates.....4 grams

Protein.....25 grams

Fat.....17 grams

Fibre.....0 grams

Sugar.....3 grams

Salt.....3.34 grams

Stuffed Avocados with Crab and Basil

204 calories per serving

Serves 4

Ingredients

White crabmeat.....100 grams, flaked

Fresh basil.....1 handful, chopped – save some whole leaves for garnish

Avocados.....2 halved

Dijon mustard.....1 teaspoon

Olive oil.....2 tablespoons

Red chilli.....1 chopped and seeded

Salt and pepper

Directions

Flake the crabmeat in a bowl. Add olive oil, mustard, salt, and pepper.

Cut the avocados in half, remove the pit and fill each cavity with a quarter of the crab mixture.

Sprinkle the basil and chili on the avocado and around the plate. Serve.

Nutrition per serving

Calories.....204

Carbohydrates.....2 grams

Protein.....6 grams

Fat.....19 grams

Fibre.....2 grams

Sugar.....1 gram

Salt.....0.41 grams

Italian Beef Stew

225 calories per serving

Serves 4

Ingredients

Beef steak.....300 grams, thinly sliced

Chopped tomatoes.....400 grams

Yellow pepper.....1 thinly sliced

Yellow onion.....1 sliced

Rosemary.....1 sprig, chopped

Garlic.....1 clove, chopped

Black olives.....1/2 cup, pitted and sliced

Olive oil.....2 tablespoons

Salt.....to taste

Directions

Heat the oil in a saucepan over medium heat. Add the garlic and onion and cook until soft.

Add the beef strips, yellow pepper, rosemary and tomatoes and bring to a boil.

Lower the heat and simmer for about 15 minutes until the meat has cooked through. Add some boiling water through the cooking process if needed.

Add the olives and cook for another couple minutes. Season with salt then serve.

Nutrition per serving

Calories.....225

Carbohydrates.....7 grams

Protein.....25 grams

Fat.....11 grams

Fibre.....2 grams

Sugar.....6 grams

Salt.....0.87 grams

Peanutty Chicken Curry

358 calories per serving

Serves 4

Ingredients

Boneless, skinless chicken breasts.....4 cut into chunks

Peanut butter.....5 tablespoons

Chicken stock.....6 ounces

Greek yogurt.....150 grams, plain

Cilantro.....1 bunch, chopped

Fresh ginger.....2 inches, chopped

Garlic.....2 cloves

Red chili.....1 large, seeded and sliced

Sunflower oil.....1 tablespoon

Directions

Place the chili, garlic, ginger, and one third of the cilantro in a food processor. Process the ingredients until you get a thick paste.

Heat the oil in a pan then lightly brown the chicken, about 1 minute. Add the chili garlic paste and stir. Add the peanut butter, yogurt, and chicken stock. Cook until the chicken has cooked through and the sauce has become thick.

Stir in the remaining cilantro. Serve.

Nutrition per serving

Calories.....358

Carbohydrates.....4 grams

Protein.....43 grams

Fat.....18.9 grams

Fibre.....1 gram

Sugar.....3 grams

Salt.....0.66 grams

Tuna Steaks with Cucumber Tomato Relish

271 calories per serving

Serves 4

Ingredients

Tuna steaks.....4 – 5 ounce tuna steaks

Olive oil.....6 tablespoons, divided

For the relish:

Tomato.....1 medium, chopped

Green onions.....2 chopped

Cucumber.....1/2 seeded and finely diced

Fresh parsley.....2 tablespoons, chopped

Lime.....1 tablespoon of lime juice

Red chili.....1/2 large seeded and chopped

Salt and pepper

Directions

Put the tuna steaks and 3 tablespoons of olive oil together in a Ziploc bag and rub together. Set aside.

For the relish, combine all the relish ingredients together in a bowl and mix. Set aside.

Heat the remaining 3 tablespoons of olive oil on a pan and cook the steaks for 2 minutes per side depending on thickness. Tuna steaks are best served slightly pink. Remove the steaks and let them rest for 5 minutes. Plate the steaks then spoon the relish over top and serve.

Nutrition per serving

Calories.....271

Carbohydrates.....2 grams

Protein.....34 grams

Fat.....14 grams

Fibre.....1 gram

Sugar.....0 grams

Salt.....0.18 grams

King Prawn Pad Thai

362 calories per serving

Serves 4

Ingredients

Rice noodles.....250 grams

Raw king prawns.....250 grams, peeled

Bean sprouts.....1 handful

Baby bok choy.....4 shredded

Green onions.....6 sliced

Fresh ginger.....1 teaspoon, chopped

Eggs.....4 beaten

Low sodium soy sauce.....1 teaspoon

Sunflower oil.....3 tablespoons, divided

Sweet chili sauce.....to serve

Directions

In a bowl, pour enough boiling water over the noodles to cover them. Let them cook in the bowl for 10 minutes. Drain.

Heat 1 tablespoon of oil in a pan. Add the prawns and ginger. Cook over high heat for 2 minutes. Transfer the prawns and ginger to a bowl.

Heat the pan again with 1 tablespoon of oil. Add the eggs. Swirl them around to coat the pan. Cook until the eggs have set. Take them out of the pan and roughly slice them. Set aside. Heat the remaining oil in the pan. Add bok choy, green onions, and bean sprouts. Cook for 2 minutes. Add the prawns and ginger mix, eggs, noodles, and soy sauce to the pan and combine. Serve with two tablespoons of sweet chili sauce per serving.

Nutrition per serving

Calories.....362

Carbohydrates.....44 grams

Protein.....21 grams

Fat.....1 gram

Fibre.....4 grams

Sugar.....2 grams

Salt.....0.82 grams

Sesame Ginger Shiitake Mushrooms with Egg Noodles

225 calories per serving

Serves 8

Ingredients

Fresh shiitake mushrooms.....300 grams, sliced

Medium dried egg noodles.....375 grams

Green onions.....8 cut into thirds and sliced lengthwise

Oyster sauce.....2 tablespoons

Sesame oil.....4 tablespoon, divided

Fresh ginger.....4 inches, grated

Low sodium soy sauce.....2 tablespoons

Peanut oil.....2 tablespoons

Directions

Cook the noodles then toss them with 2 tablespoons of sesame oil.

Heat the peanut oil in a wok on high heat. Add the ginger then add the mushrooms along with a splash of water. Cook for 1 minute. Add the noodles and cook for 2 minutes then add the green onions, soy sauce, oyster sauce, and the remaining 2 tablespoons of sesame oil. Serve.

Nutrition per serving

Calories.....225

Carbohydrates.....35 grams

Protein.....7 grams

Fat.....8 grams

Fibre.....2 grams

Sugar.....2 grams

Salt.....1.36 grams

Steak with Zesty Herb Sauce

303 calories per serving

Serves 2

Ingredients

Sirloin steaks.....2 – 125 grams each

Fresh parsley.....1 small bunch, chopped

Shallot.....1 chopped

Garlic.....2 cloves

Juice of ½ a lemon

Red wine vinegar.....2 tablespoons

Oregano.....1/2 teaspoon, dried

Chili flakes.....1/2 teaspoon

Olive oil.....6 tablespoons, divided

Salt and pepper.....to taste

Directions

Mix the oregano, garlic, chili flakes, shallot, parsley, lemon juice, red wine vinegar, and 3 tablespoons olive oil together in a food processor.

Work the remaining oil into the steaks and season with salt and pepper. Heat a pan and cook the steaks for 2 minutes per side. Remove from pan and let the steaks rest.

Top the steaks with the oregano garlic mixture. Serve.

Nutrition per serving

Calories.....303

Carbohydrates.....1 gram

Protein.....30 grams

Fat.....20 grams

Fibre.....1 gram

Sugar.....1 gram

Salt.....0.3 grams

Crab and Avocado Salad

419 calories per serving

Serves 4

Ingredients

Crabmeat.....450 grams (mix of white and brown meat)

Cherry tomatoes.....12

Avocado.....1 cut lengthwise

Crème Fraîche.....150 ml

Rocket leaf lettuce.....110 gram bag, washed

Juice of 1 lemon

Olive oil.....3 tablespoons

Salt.....to taste

Directions

Mix the crabmeat, crème fraîche, salt, and half the lemon juice together until smooth. Set aside.

Combine the lettuce, avocado and tomatoes in a large bowl. Squeeze the remaining lemon juice over the salad along with the olive oil.

Plate the salad and top with the crabmeat mixture. Serve.

Nutrition per serving

Calories.....419

Carbohydrates.....48 grams

Protein.....25 grams

Fat.....34 grams

Fibre.....3 grams

Sugar.....2 grams

Salt.....1.24 grams

Asian Salmon and Broccoli Bake

310 calories per serving

Serves 4

Ingredients

Salmon fillets.....4 fillets with skin

Broccoli.....1 head, florets only

Green onions.....1 small bunch

Low sodium soy sauce.....2 tablespoons

Juice of ½ lemon.....quarter the other half

Directions

Preheat the oven to 200 degrees. Place the salmon in a roasting tin leaving space between each fillet.

Arrange the broccoli in the roasting tin alongside the salmon. Pour the lemon juice over the salmon and broccoli and add lemon quarters to the roasting tin.

Top with half the green onions and drizzle lightly with olive oil. Cook in the oven for 15 minutes.

Remove from the oven and sprinkle with soy sauce then return to oven for another 4 minutes. Sprinkle with the remaining green onions. Serve.

Nutrition per serving

Calories.....310

Carbohydrates.....3 grams

Protein.....35 grams

Fat.....17 grams

Fibre.....4 grams

Sugar.....3 grams

Salt.....1.6 grams

Beef and Oyster Sauce Stir-Fry

286 calories per serving

Serves 4

Ingredients

Lean beef steak.....450 grams, cut into slices, about 5 cm long

Rice wine or dry sherry.....1 tablespoon

Oyster sauce.....3 tablespoons

Low sodium soy sauce.....1 tablespoon

Green pepper.....1 diced

Red pepper.....1 diced

Sesame oil.....2 tablespoons

Corn flour.....2 tablespoons

Peanut oil.....3 tablespoons

Green onions.....2 finely chopped for garnish

Directions

Place the beef steak in a bowl and mix together with soy sauce, rice wine, or sherry, sesame oil and corn flour. Marinate for 15 minutes.

Heat the peanut oil in a wok. Add the beef steak and stir-fry until lightly brown. Remove the meat. Discard the oil in the wok and wipe the wok clean.

Reheat the wok and add the green and red pepper. Cook for 3 minutes or until soft. Add the oyster sauce and simmer. Return the beef steak to the wok and stir together. Transfer the contents of the wok to a serving platter and top with green onions. Serve.

Nutrition per serving

Calories.....286

Carbohydrates.....8 grams

Protein.....25 grams

Fat.....17 grams

Fibre.....2 grams

Sugar.....4 grams

Salt.....2 grams

Pineapple Curry with Turkey Meatballs

258 calories per serving

Serves 4

Ingredients

Ground turkey.....1 pound, 454 grams

Pineapple chunks in juice.....1 – 10 ounce can drained, reserve the juice

Korma paste.....4 tablespoons (Korma paste is a mild curry paste)

Low-fat coconut milk.....400 ml can

Cilantro.....1 small bunch, chopped

Almonds.....6 tablespoons, crushed

Yellow onion.....1 chopped

Fresh ginger.....2 inches grated

Garlic.....2 cloves

Vegetable oil.....1 tablespoon

Basmati rice.....to serve

Salt and pepper

Directions

Strain the pineapples and reserve the juice. From the reserved juice keep 2 tablespoons of juice separate. Season the ground turkey with salt and pepper and shape into mini meatballs. Heat the oil in a pan and add the meatballs. Cook until brown. In a food processor blend the garlic, ginger, onion, cilantro, and the 2 tablespoons of pineapple juice. Move the meatballs to one side of the pan and add the garlic blend. Cook until soft. Add korma paste and stir together with the meatballs. Add the crushed almonds, pineapple chunks, coconut milk, pineapple juice, salt, and pepper. Simmer uncovered for 10 minutes. Serve.

Nutrition per serving

Calories.....258

Carbohydrates.....7 grams

Protein.....35 grams

Fat.....11 grams

Fibre.....2 grams

Sugar.....5 grams

Salt.....0.88 grams

Stuffed Zucchini Rolls

49 calories per roll

Makes 24 rolls

Ingredients

Zucchini.....4 small sliced lengthwise into 24 long strips to wrap

Ricotta cheese.....250 grams

Fresh basil.....1 handful, chopped

Pine nuts.....1 handful, toasted

Balsamic vinegar.....to drizzle

Juice of 1 lemon

Olive oil.....to drizzle

Salt and pepper

Directions

Preheat the oven to 200 degrees. Cut the ends off the zucchini. Use a mandolin to slice the zucchini lengthwise into ¼ inch slices.

Lay the zucchini strips down on a greased baking sheet without overlapping them. Lightly drizzle some oil and balsamic vinegar over the zucchini strips. Sprinkle with a little more oil and balsamic vinegar. Cover and marinate in the fridge for 15 minutes. Remove from fridge and place the zucchini in the oven. Cook for 4 minutes until the zucchini is soft enough to roll.

Mix the ricotta cheese together with the lemon juice, salt, basil, and pine nuts. Place the ricotta mixture on one end of a zucchini strip and roll it up. Repeat this for all 24 zucchini strips.

Arrange the zucchini rolls upright on a plate and season with salt and pepper. Drizzle with more oil and balsamic vinegar. Serve.

Nutrition per serving

Calories.....49

Carbohydrates.....1 gram

Protein.....2 grams

Fat.....5 grams

Fibre.....0 grams

Sugar.....1 gram

Salt.....0.03 grams

Crème Fraîche Herb Chicken

298 calories per serving

Serves 5

Ingredients

Skinless, boneless chicken thighs.....750 grams, cut into large chunks

Crème Fraîche.....175 grams, half-fat

Apple cider vinegar.....14 ounces

Fresh parsley.....1 small handful, chopped

Fresh thyme.....1 tablespoon, leaves picked

Whole grain mustard.....2 tablespoons

Yellow onions.....2 sliced

Garlic.....3 cloves

Olive oil.....1 tablespoon

Steamed broccoli to serve

Salt and pepper

Directions

Heat the oil in a pan (that has a lid). Cook the chicken for 3 minutes on each side until brown. Remove from heat with a slotted spoon then add the onions and garlic to the pan. Cook for 3 minutes. Add the apple cider vinegar and bring to boil. Return the chicken to the pan. Cover with lid and simmer for 10 minutes.

Remove the lid and add the mustard, crème fraîche, and herbs. Bring to a mild boil and season with salt and pepper. Serve with steamed broccoli.

Nutrition per serving

Calories.....298

Carbohydrates.....8 grams

Protein.....34 grams

Fat.....12 grams

Fibre.....2 grams

Sugar.....6 grams

Salt.....0.6 grams

Sweet Steak with Barbecue Sauce

358 calories per serving

Serves 4

Ingredients

Lamb or beef steaks.....4 – 4 ounce steaks

White onion.....1 chopped

Worcestershire sauce.....3 tablespoons

Red wine vinegar.....2 tablespoons

Brown sugar.....2 tablespoon

Ketchup.....150 ml

Sunflower oil.....6 tablespoon

Salt and pepper

Directions

Heat a pan with oil on medium heat. Brush the steaks with 3 tablespoons of oil and season with salt and pepper on both sides. Place them on the pan and cook until tender.

To make the sauce, heat the remaining oil in a pan and add the onion. Cook until soft. Add all the remaining ingredients and simmer for 5 minutes.

Plate the steaks and serve with the sauce drizzled over top.

Nutrition per serving

Calories.....358

Carbohydrates.....23 grams

Protein.....38 grams

Fat.....14 grams

Fibre.....1 gram

Sugar.....21 grams

Salt.....2.13 grams

Spaghetti with Spanish Flavors

444 calories per serving

Serves 4

Ingredients

Chorizo sausage.....80 grams, sliced

Spaghetti noodles.....300 grams

Roasted red peppers.....1 – 7 ounce jar, chopped

Flat leaf parsley.....1 handful, chopped

Fresh parmesan.....100 grams plus extra to serve

Olive oil.....2 tablespoons

Salt and pepper

Directions

Cook the spaghetti according to package directions. Reserve half a cup of pasta water when draining.

Heat the oil in a frying pan and add chorizo, roasted red peppers, salt, and pepper. Cook for about 2 minutes. Add spaghetti, parsley, and parmesan to the pan along with the half cup of reserved pasta water.

Serve with extra parmesan on the table.

Nutrition per serving

Calories....444

Carbohydrates.....46 grams

Protein.....18 grams

Fat.....22 grams

Fibre.....3 grams

Sugar.....0 grams

Salt.....2.21 grams

Pork 'n Fruit Steaks

304 calories per serving

Serves 4

Ingredients

Boneless pork loin steaks.....4 steaks trimmed of fat

Chicken stock.....200 ml

Chinese five-spice powder.....2 teaspoons

Red apples.....4 cored and diced

Red currant jelly.....2 tablespoons

Red wine vinegar.....1 tablespoon

Red onion.....1 cut into wedges

Sunflower oil.....4 tablespoons, divided

Directions

Season the pork steaks with Chinese five-spice powder.

Heat 2 tablespoons of oil in a frying pan. Fry the pork for 3 minutes per side until brown. Transfer to a plate.

Heat the remaining oil along with onion wedges for about 2 minutes. Add the apples and cook for 3 minutes. Add the jelly, red wine vinegar, and chicken stock. Bring to a boil and simmer uncovered for 8 minutes until the sauce is syrupy. Place the pork into the sauce turning each piece to glaze.

Nutrition per serving

Calories....304

Carbohydrates.....25 grams

Protein.....33 grams

Fat.....9 grams

Fibre.....38 grams

Sugar.....24 grams

Salt.....0.79 grams

Lime and Ginger Salmon

354 calories per serving

Serves 2

Ingredients

Skinless salmon fillets.....2

Chicken stock.....4 ounces

Baby corn.....140 grams, halved

Baby Chinese cabbage.....4 chopped

Thin stemmed broccoli.....200 grams

Fresh ginger.....2 inches, grated

Garlic.....2 cloves, crushed

Low sodium soy sauce.....2 tablespoons

Rice wine vinegar.....2 tablespoons

Green onions.....3 chopped

Juice of 2 limes

Cooking spray

Pepper

Directions

Heat the oven to 350 degrees.

Mix the ginger, garlic, soy sauce, rice wine vinegar, lime juice, and pepper together in a bowl. Pour half over the salmon to marinate for 10 minutes. Reserve the marinade.

Place salmon fillets on a baking tray and bake for 5 minutes per side. Heat a wok with the reserved marinade and the chicken stock. Add baby corn, broccoli and stir-fry for 5 minutes. Add Chinese cabbage and cook for 2 minutes. Plate the vegetables. Place the salmon on top of the vegetables. Pour the sauce over the salmon. Sprinkle with green onions.

Nutrition per serving

Calories....354

Carbohydrates.....11 grams

Protein.....38 grams

Fat.....18 grams

Fibre.....6 grams

Sugar.....7 grams

Salt.....1.4 grams

Minty Turkey and Bulgur

224 calories per roll

Serves 2

Ingredients

Turkey breast.....200 grams, diced

Whole grain bulgur wheat.....50 grams

Plain Greek yogurt.....2 tablespoons

Tomatoes.....2 chopped

English long cucumber.....1/2 diced

Fresh parsley.....2 tablespoons, chopped

Fresh mint.....2 tablespoons, chopped

Red onion.....1 small, finely chopped

Garlic.....2 cloves, crushed

Smoked paprika.....1/2 teaspoon

Juice of 1 lemon, divided

Directions

Cook the bulgur according to package directions then add the tomatoes, cucumber, parsley, mint, red onion, and half the lemon juice. Stir.

Line a baking tray with tin foil. Mix the yogurt, paprika, remaining half of lemon juice, and garlic together then add the turkey. Stir together then arrange on the tray.

Bake the turkey mix for 7 minutes. Serve hot or cold with bulgur.

Nutrition per serving

Calories....224

Carbohydrates.....24 grams

Protein.....27 grams

Fat.....2 grams

Fibre.....2 grams

Sugar.....5 grams

Salt.....0.2 grams

Pork in Chunky Marmalade Sauce

335 calories per serving

Serves 4

Ingredients

Pork steaks.....4 steaks, about ¾ inch thick

Chicken stock.....8 ounces

Chunky marmalade.....4 tablespoons

Fresh thyme.....1 tablespoon

Garlic.....3 cloves, sliced

Olive oil.....1 tablespoon

Steamed spinach, peas, and carrots.....to serve

Salt and pepper

Directions

Season the pork with salt and pepper.

Heat the olive oil in a pan. Add garlic then pork and cook for 6 minutes per side until golden. Remove pork and let it rest on a warm plate.

Mix the marmalade and thyme together in a bowl.

Add the chicken stock and marmalade mixture to the pan. Heat until it bubbles to make a sauce. Thicken with cornstarch if needed. Return the pork to the pan and coat.

Serve with steamed spinach, peas, and carrots.

Nutrition per serving

Calories....335

Carbohydrates.....14 grams

Protein.....42 grams

Fat.....13 grams

Fibre.....0.2 grams

Sugar.....13 grams

Salt.....0.2 grams

Crab Tostadas with Pickled Onion and Lime

394 calories per serving

Serves 2

Ingredients

White crabmeat.....170 grams, drained

Avocado.....1 mashed

Red onion.....1 sliced into rings

Whole wheat tortillas.....2

Mixed salad leaves.....1 handful

Garlic.....2 cloves, crushed

Green onions.....2 finely sliced

Red chili.....1 seeded and chopped

Juice of 2 limes, keep the juice of each lime separate

1 lime......for wedges to serve

Sugar.....pinch

Salt and pepper

Directions

Mix the red onion, juice of one lime, a pinch of salt and sugar together in a bowl. Set aside to soften.

Mix the crabmeat, green onions, and half the red chili together. Season with pepper and set aside.

Mix the avocado together with garlic, salt, and remaining lime juice and chili. The avocado can be smooth or chunky....your choice. Toast the tortillas in a toaster for 1 minute. Put the tortillas on 2 plates and top with mixed salad leaves, mashed avocado, crabmeat, and pickled onion. Serve with lime wedges.

Nutrition per serving

Calories....394

Carbohydrates.....27 grams

Protein.....22 grams

Fat.....19 grams

Fibre.....6 grams

Sugar.....5 grams

Salt.....1.1 grams

Cranberry Chicken Salad

190 calories per serving

Serves 4

Ingredients

Skinless, boneless chicken breast.....2 (4 ounces each), sliced to make 4 thin breasts

Cucumber.....1/2 seeded and sliced

Dried cranberries.....25 grams

Red onion.....2 thinly sliced

Mixed salad leaves.....200 grams

Cranberry sauce.....3 ounces

Juice of 1 lime

Olive oil.....6 tablespoons, divided

Water.....2 tablespoons

Salt and pepper

Directions

Rub 3 tablespoons of olive oil on the chicken and season with salt and pepper.

Heat 3 tablespoons of oil on a pan then fry the red onion. Add the chicken and cook for about 3 minutes per side. Set aside.

Remove the chicken and slice. Keep the pan warm and add the cranberry sauce, dried cranberries, water, and lime juice to the chicken drippings and onions.

In a salad bowl, combine the mixed salad leaves, cucumber, chicken slices, and cranberry dressing. Serve immediately.

Nutrition per serving

Calories....190

Carbohydrates.....19 grams

Protein.....18 grams

Fat.....5 grams

Fibre.....2 grams

Sugar.....17 grams

Salt.....0.12 grams

Smoked Salmon with Green Beans and Chives

488 calories per serving

Serves 2

Ingredients

Smoked salmon.....250 grams

Green beans.....200 grams

New potatoes.....150 grams, halved

Olive oil.....2 tablespoons

For the dressing:

White wine vinegar.....2 tablespoons

Dijon mustard.....1 teaspoon

Fresh chives......1 handful

Vegetable oil.....2 tablespoons

Sugar.....1 teaspoon

Directions

Mix all the dressing ingredients together in a bowl.

Cook the potatoes in boiling water for 8 minutes. Add the green beans to the boiling water and cook for another 4 minutes until soft. Drain. Add the potatoes and green beans to the mustard dressing. Toss.

Heat 2 tablespoons of olive oil in a pan then add the salmon. Cook for 3 minutes per side. Plate the potatoes and beans and top with salmon.

Nutrition per serving

Calories....488

Carbohydrates.....34 grams

Protein.....24 grams

Fat.....29 grams

Fibre.....4 grams

Sugar.....3 grams

Salt.....3.83 grams

Garam Masala Chicken with Mango Salsa

262 calories per serving

Serves 4

Ingredients

Skinless, boneless chicken breasts.....4 sliced

Garam masala.....1 tablespoon

Plain Greek yogurt.....4 tablespoons

Mango.....1 large, cut into slim wedges

Long English cucumber.....1/2 cut lengthwise

Red onion.....1/2 sliced

Cilantro.....1 handful

Lime.....1 juice and zest, keep the zest separate from the juice

Olive oil.....2 tablespoons

Naan bread.....to serve

Salt.....to taste

Directions

Heat the olive oil in a pan. Add the chicken, garam masala, and salt. Cook for 6 minutes per side. Slice the chicken diagonally.

Toss the mango, cucumber, red onion, cilantro, and lime juice together and plate.

Mix the yogurt together with the lime zest and salt, and serve alongside the salad.

Place the chicken alongside the salad and serve.

Nutrition per serving

Calories....262

Carbohydrates.....16 grams

Protein.....36 grams

Fat.....7 grams

Fibre.....3 grams

Sugar.....0 grams

Salt.....0.25 grams

Prawn Fajitas with Creamy Avocado Sauce

320 calories per serving

Serves 2

Ingredients

Large raw prawns.....225 grams

Sour cream.....1 heaping tablespoon

Avocado.....1 roughly chopped

Red pepper.....1 seeded and sliced

Cilantro.....1 small bunch, chopped

Garlic.....6 cloves, crushed

Red chili.....1 seeded and chopped

Juice of 2 limes

Lime.....1 for wedges to serve

Whole wheat tortillas.....4

Olive oil.....1 tablespoon

A large handful of mixed salad leaves to serve

Salt.....to taste

Directions

Mix half the garlic, half the lime juice, half the chili, half the cilantro, and salt together in a bowl. Add the prawns and mix. Place the avocado, salt, remaining chili, garlic, lime juice, and sour cream together in a food processor. Stir in the remaining cilantro.

Heat the oil in a pan and cook the red pepper until soft. Add the prawn mixture and fry for 1 minute each side. Divide the prawn and red pepper mixture between four tortillas. Roll the tortillas with the mixture and serve with the salad leaves and avocado cream. Include lime wedges on side.

Nutrition per serving

Calories....320

Carbohydrates.....8 grams

Protein.....23 grams

Fat.....22 grams

Fibre.....5 grams

Sugar.....6 grams

Salt.....0.6 grams

Cilantro Chicken Korma

376 calories per serving

Serves 4

Ingredients

Skinless, boneless chicken breasts.....4 (approx. 4 ounces each) cut into bite-sized pieces

Chicken stock.....12 ounces

Korma paste.....4 tablespoons (Korma paste is a mild curry paste)

Plain Greek yogurt.....150 grams

Cilantro.....1/2 a small bunch, chopped

Yellow onion.....1 chopped

Sultana raisins.....4 tablespoons

Ground almonds.....2 tablespoons

Fresh ginger.....2 inches, grated

Garlic.....2 cloves, chopped

Water.....4 tablespoons

Sugar.....1/4 teaspoon

Salt.....to taste

Directions

Place the ginger, garlic, and onion in a food processor and mix together to form a paste. Remove and place in a heated pan along with 4 tablespoons of water. Cook for 5 minutes. Add the korma paste and cook for another 2 minutes.

Place the chicken into the pan with the sauce. Add ground almonds, chicken stock, sultana raisins, and sugar. Mix. Cover and simmer for 10 minutes.

Remove from heat and stir in the yogurt and salt. Top with cilantro. Serve.

Nutrition per serving

Calories....376

Carbohydrates.....28 grams

Protein.....40 grams

Fat.....11 grams

Fibre.....3 grams

Sugar.....26 grams

Salt.....1.1 grams

Smoked Salmon and Grapefruit Fennel Salad

291 calories per serving

Serves 4

Ingredients

Smoked salmon fillets.....4 fillets

Grapefruit.....2 (white or pink, your choice) segmented, keep juice separate

Watercress.....100 gram bag

Fennel bulb.....1 large, sliced

Fennel seeds.....2 teaspoons, crushed

Red onion.....1 sliced

For the dressing:

Wholegrain mustard.....2 tablespoons

Honey.....2 teaspoons

Olive oil.....2 tablespoons

Salt.....to taste

Directions

Place the segmented grapefruit in a bowl. Squeeze the grapefruit juice into a separate bowl.

To make the dressing, mix the honey, mustard, and olive oil together with the grapefruit juice. Season to taste.

Mix the grapefruit segments with red onion, watercress, fennel bulb, and half the dressing.

Plate the grapefruit and flake the salmon over top. Drizzle with remaining dressing then top with crushed fennel seeds.

Nutrition per serving

Calories....291

Carbohydrates.....11 grams

Protein.....23 grams

Fat.....18 grams

Fibre.....4 grams

Sugar.....11 grams

Salt.....1.4 grams

Sesame Basil Chicken Salad

300 calories per serving

Serves 2

Ingredients

Skinless, boneless chicken breasts.....2 (4 ounce pieces), sliced

Carrot.....1 large, sliced into sticks

Cherry tomatoes.....140 grams, halved

Fresh basil.....1 handful, chopped

Mixed salad leaves.....100 grams

Sesame seeds.....1 teaspoon, toasted

Cilantro.....1 small bunch, chopped

Green onions.....4 finely sliced

Olive oil....2 tablespoons

Salt and pepper

For the dressing:

Fish sauce.....3 teaspoon

Sesame oil.....3 teaspoon

Sweet chili sauce.....4 teaspoons

Juice of 1 lime

Directions

Mix the dressing ingredients together in a bowl and set aside.

Heat the oil on a pan. Season the chicken with salt and pepper then add it to the pan and cook through. Slice the chicken then toss it with the dressing. Add basil, carrots, tomatoes, cilantro, and green onions to the chicken mix and toss.

Plate the mixed salad leaves and top with chicken dressing mixture. Sprinkle with sesame seeds.

Nutrition per serving

Calories....300

Carbohydrates.....14 grams

Protein.....44 grams

Fat.....7 grams

Fibre.....7 grams

Sugar.....12 grams

Salt.....1 gram

Roasted Carrot, Feta and Mixed Seeds Salad

221 calories per serving

Serves 2

Ingredients

Carrots.....300 grams, sliced into thin rounds

Feta cheese.....2 tablespoons

Spinach leaves.....2 large handfuls

Red wine vinegar.....2 tablespoons

Caraway seeds.....1 teaspoon

Pumpkin seeds.....1 tablespoon

Sunflower seeds.....1 tablespoon

Zest of 1 orange

Olive oil.....2 teaspoons, divided

Salt.....to taste

Directions

Heat the oven to 250 degrees.

Boil the carrots until soft. Drain then toss with the caraway seeds and place onto a baking pan along with 1 teaspoon of olive oil, orange zest, and salt. Roast for 20 minutes until soft.

Segment the zested orange over a bowl. Catch any orange juice. Add the remaining oil to the bowl with red wine vinegar, seeds, and salt. Stir.

Combine the orange mix with the spinach leaves and roasted carrots.

Plate and top with feta cheese.

Nutrition per serving

Calories....221

Carbohydrates.....22 grams

Protein.....9 grams

Fat.....12 grams

Fibre.....6 grams

Sugar.....19 grams

Salt.....1.2 grams

Vegetable Tempura

471 calories per serving

Serves 4

Ingredients

Zucchini.....150 grams, cut into bite-sized pieces

Broccoli florets.....150 grams

Mushrooms.....150 grams, halved

Red pepper.....150 grams, cut into bite-sized pieces

Aubergine.....150 grams, cut into bite-sized pieces

Carrot.....150 grams, sliced

Sunflower oil.....for deep frying

For the dipping sauce:

Low sodium soy sauce.....3 tablespoons

Dry sherry.....3 tablespoons

Sugar.....1 tablespoon

Lemon.....1 zest only

Tempura batter:

Flour.....3 ounces

Corn flour.....1 tablespoon

Sea salt.....1/2 teaspoon

Mineral water.....7 ounces

Ice cubes.....8

Directions

Tempura batter

Prepare the tempura batter just before using. Combine both flour and corn flour with sea salt and mix. Whisk in the mineral water and ice cubes. Don't over beat and don't worry if it's lumpy. When using the batter make sure the batter is ice cold and the oil hot in order to get a crispy exterior on each vegetable.

Tempura dipping sauce

Combine all of the dipping sauce ingredients together. Set aside.

Vegetable tempura

Heat the oven to 250 degrees. Mix the sauce ingredients together in a bowl. Set aside.

Make the tempura batter.

Heat a large wok that is 1/3 full of oil. When the oil is very hot dip a vegetable into some batter then place it into the hot oil. Don't cook too many vegetables at once. After about 2 minutes of frying each vegetable remove from oil with a slotted spoon and place on a paper towel that you have laid out on a plate.

Serve with the dipping sauce.

Nutrition per serving

Calories....471

Carbohydrates.....33 grams

Protein.....5 grams

Fat.....35 grams

Fibre.....4 grams

Sugar.....4 grams

Salt.....2.08 grams

Leftover Turkey and Ham Noodle Medley

476 calories per serving

Serves 4

Ingredients

Leftover turkey meat.....250 grams, shredded

Leftover ham.....140 grams, diced

Rice noodles.....200 grams

Bean sprouts.....200 grams

Red peppers.....2 seeded and sliced

Fresh ginger.....2 inches, minced

Garlic.....4 cloves, chopped

Green onions.....6 finely sliced

Curry powder.....3 tablespoons

Sesame oil.....2 tablespoons, divided

Eggs.....2 beaten

Turmeric.....1 teaspoon

Low sodium soy sauce.....4 tablespoons, divided

Dry sherry.....2 tablespoons

Sugar.....1 tablespoon

Vegetable oil.....2 tablespoons, divided

Cilantro.....1 small bunch, chopped to serve

Salt.....to taste

Directions

Place the rice noodles in a bowl and cover with boiling water. Drain when the noodles are tender. Toss the noodles with 1 tablespoon of sesame oil. Set aside.

Beat the eggs with the remaining sesame oil and salt. Set aside.

Heat one tablespoon of vegetable oil in a wok. Add the eggs and swirl to cover the bottom of the wok and form an omelet. Cook until eggs have set. Remove and transfer to plate.

Reheat the wok with the remaining oil and add the garlic and ginger. Add the vegetables and fry for 2 minutes then add the ham and turkey. Cook until the vegetables are soft and the meat has been warmed through. Remove the vegetables and meat from the wok. Cover and keep warm.

Place the noodles, curry powder, turmeric, two tablespoons soy sauce, sherry, and sugar in the wok and cook for 2 minutes.

Slice the omelet and add it to the noodles. Add the cilantro to noodles along with the remaining soy sauce.

Plate the noodles and top with the vegetable, ham, and turkey mixture. Serve.

Nutrition per serving

Calories....476

Carbohydrates.....36 grams

Protein.....50 grams

Fat.....13 grams

Fibre.....4 grams

Sugar.....8 grams

Salt.....3 grams

Conclusion

Eating healthy is a lifestyle but in order to make it something you naturally do it will take some discipline and hard work at first. Stick with it! I'm proof that you can have anything that you are determined to get.

I hope you enjoy the recipes and use them to make your fast days tastier and easier!

Reviews

If you received value from this book please consider posting a review on Amazon. Even a one or two line review is helpful and much appreciated!

Other Books by Gina Crawford

5:2 Diet for Beginners

Mediterranean Diet for Beginners

Mediterranean Diet Recipes

DASH Diet for Beginners

DASH Diet Recipes

Sugar Detox for Beginners

Sugar Free Recipes

Paleo for Beginners

About the Author

Gina Crawford is a health and "all things natural" enthusiast and the author of several diet and health related books. After spending years of her life overweight, exhausted, and unhappy Gina made a quality decision to turn her life around. She began researching everything she could on diet, health, weight loss, and transforming her life. With dedication and perseverance she achieved her goal weight and improved her health so much that her energy level and zest for life skyrocketed. She is now on a mission to share what she learned in a concise, easy to understand, to the point kind of way that allows others to achieve maximum results in a short amount of time. Helping people live better, healthier, more passionate lives is her ultimate desire.

Made in the USA
Middletown, DE
13 March 2017